How To Give Your Wife An Amazing Pussy Massage

A Step-By-Step Guide

Thomas Kaine

Table Of Contents

A real truth is that physical touch between a couple really deepens the level of romance and emotional intimacy in the couple's relationship. So, what better way to maximize that physical touch than with an erotic pussy massage?

This is not just ANY type of body massage, but a massage that actually stimulates her genitals.

Yes, you heard me right sir! We're talking about an erotic genital massage, with just your fingers folks! A pussy massage is actually a tantric practice that boosts and couples intimacy and connects you and your partner emotionally, physically, and yes sensually. It's not simply to stimulate her genitals, like an anal massage, for example.

However, it's also not just about placing your hands inside her pussy and massaging her randomly for ten seconds. There are some very important things you should know first.

This book will guide you step by step on how to give a pussy massage your lover will truly love.

Chapter 1

What Actually Is A Pussy Massage?

A pussy massage is also called a yoni massage.

It's a type of sensual massage that actually focuses on the woman's vagina, and not necessarily just for foreplay or sex. *(I mean, it could lead to those things, but it's not the end goal most of the time.)*

Usually, it's performed by some type of a professional therapist or masseuse specializing in giving a yoni massage. But you can also perform this very intimate massage as an **erotic** full-body massage to really pleasure your partner.

Yoni is a Sanskrit word that means a vagina.

In translation, it means "a sacred space." That means a yoni massage or pussy massage esteems the vagina as a most sacred part of her body that totally deserves adoration and honor.

Giving a pussy massage to your girl goes her more than just a regular body massage.

The truth is this type of massage can actually give her some deep relaxation and physical pleasure like she has never had before. Yes, a pussy massage is that special.

And even more than that, it could also be a healing true experience for her and an opportunity to build a stronger connection in your relationship—physically, emotionally, and yes even sexually.

Here are more reasons why you should try a pussy massage with your wife today:

It helps her be more in tune with her own body

As the receiver of the massage, it helps your wife relax and feel more comfortable and in tune with her body. For some reason most women actually hate their body. There is always something wrong with it. During other sexual acts a couple does in the bedroom, each person is somewhat required to give and receive. But during a pussy massage, she's not required to give back anything to her lover. Instead, she can relish the sensations and better understand what feels good to her.

It also allows her to relax

Stress for a lady can lead to her having a low sex drive. It's difficult for most women to be in the mood for sex when her body is always tired and stressed out. A pussy massage can help her truly relax as you can knead different pressure points in her body in this region.

It also Improves your sexual relationship

As we have already mentioned, a pussy massage is a slow, sensual and methodical practice. If she's holding back from you because of a fear of intimacy and touch, this is a good practice to get her to ease into it. In addition, learning what's pleasurable for your wife is a bonding experience that could supercharge her sexual confidence.

It also supports mental healing

It's so important to be respectful toward your lover and always go slow, especially if she has any shame, sexual trauma, or negative emotions attached to her genitals. Studies have shown that most women don't like how their genitals look or smell. Even though most have never did an inspection with a mirror, they still don't like it. It's good for you as her husband to calm her tensions by telling her how beautiful her pussy looks and how awesome it smells and even tastes. I often take my fingers out of it in front of her and lick my fingers clean as I moan in pleasure. Most of the time she just smiles when I do this. I know it is assuring her that I love her pussy and think it is pretty amazing. With a pussy massage, you can learn better how to touch her and help her reprogram these experiences into positive and pleasurable feelings.

It also encourages more intense orgasms

The amazing sensations and the combination of the factors we mentioned above potentially result in a woman experiencing way more intense climaxes. The mind is a very important component for a female orgasm. Add to that the physical pleasure of the massage itself and you have a winning combination.

Chapter 2

What Are The Benefits Of A Pussy Massage?

A good pussy massage can actually become a real therapeutic experience for couples to share together. One is the giver, while the other is the receiver. This means that there is no pressure to PERFORM for a lover.

You can just take all the time you need to explore her lavish body and learn what truly feels good to her. While she can indulge in the amazing sensations she is receiving without any rush, pressure, or judgment.

With that being said, let's jump into the steps on how to give an erotic pussy massage.

Chapter 3

Preparing Yourself To Give A Pussy Massage

Prepare Your Mindset. Your role as the giver of an intimate pussy massage is VERY important in the effectiveness in the pussy massage. YOU set the tone for the massage. YOU need to make her feel safe. YOU ate responsible to build the energy during the massage session. You should make an attempt to worship her body and make her feel like a goddess. The erotic experience only becomes impactful when you are connected to her and when you can be intentional and purposeful in the act of revering her.

The Proper Mindset For You

You are to give, give, give

As the giver, you are being unconditional because you are giving her a massage without expecting anything in return. That means you also should not pressure yourself into making her orgasm—because that's NOT the goal. Also, I must tell you that I never give her a pussy massage without multiple orgasms following. After all my wife is one of those ladies who is what I call orgasmic. Or she can cum quite easily. She even cums when she is deep throating my cock.

Remind yourself that the main purpose of this erotic practice is to serve her, or heal her, and even to connect with her on a deeper level.

This goes both ways as well. Go ahead and let your partner know that she IS NOT expected to have an orgasm. Liberate her from feeling like she has any obligations to perform or give something back to you. If anything happens as a result of the pussy massage, consider it a ~BONUS~.

You should take things S-L-O-W

The key to an effective pussy massage is to be SLOW and SENSUAL. Did you her that sir, slow and sensual.

Touch her pussy as slowly and softly as you have ever done before. You should be intentional in each stroke, like it's an act of deep meditation.

Going slow allows you to explore her vaginal area like you never did before, especially when you're still starting out. This also gives you more room to wiggle on how she wants to move forward with the massage. Does she want it to turn into something more or not. She might want you to increase the pressure, intensity, or speed of your fingers. She might even ask you to insert a finger or two when she's aroused and bring her to an orgasm.

Communicate With her

Communication above all else is one of the critical aspects of giving your wife a pussy massage and any other kind of sexual act. And that's both VERBAL and NONVERBAL.

You can simply just ask her questions like "Does this feel good?" or "Do you want me to go faster or slower baby?" Let her be vocal about how she feels as well. In fact, you should encourage it.

Of course, as I said, you should be attentive to her physical cues as well. For example, she might moan or grind her hips towards your hands, that means that she likes what you are doing at that time.

If she cringes and kind of moves away from your hands, that means she didn't like it. Ask her why—*was it too sensitive?* What could you do instead that she would like?

Prepare The Space For Intimacy

You shouldn't overlook the power of creating a safe and sacred space when you are exploring a tantric practice like a pussy massage.

Your surroundings actually have a BIG impact on your sensuality and sexuality. So, you should make your space feel like a pleasure sanctuary, especially during the massage session.

Set Up A Special Space

This is so important and yet so overlooked by most people. You need to create a space that is both physically and energetically.

To do so, you should remove all clutter from the room. Throw away all the unused items, junk, and any trash that might be lying around. These things carry negative energy and remind you of the daily stresses of life that you and your lover would want to get away from for at least a few hours.

Make Sure You Have The Right Temperature

You should do you best to avoid having your room too cold. Am effective pussy massage requires your partner to go completely naked. You wouldn't want her to be shivering throughout.

A slightly too warm room is inviting for a sensual time. It also promotes relaxation on her part.
But make sure it's not too warm that you'll be dripping in sweat as you do the massage—which is physically

taxing. We have compensated for this by buying a warming massage table to do the massages on. There really isn't a chance of her getting cold as she lays on a table that is warm and you can actually regulate how warm you want to table.

Use Dim Lighting

Cool, bright lights are simply put for reading and studying. I mean, there's a reason why spas always have dim and warm lights—because *they're relaxing!* You can cover your lamps and just light a candle instead. In fact, why not light candles that have a scent to them.

Make The Space Also Smell Inviting

Doing a tantric pussy massage can heighten all the senses. That means you should include the olfactory senses as well. Scents can quickly set the mood in your space.

Still, you'd want to choose the right scents. It's nice to have calming aromatherapy, but not too calming that she'd end up falling asleep. Unfortunately, my wife has fallen asleep several times during a pussy massage. Some good scents to choose from are lavender, jasmine, citrus, rosemary, and lemon. They're relaxing but could still feel invigorating.

Prepping Your Massage Oil

You will want your hands to glide along her curves as you stroke her body with your hands when you do the massage. Too much friction could feel uncomfortable and far from relaxing. For that reason, massage oils are imperative.

There are many different types of massage oils available. The most popular ones are essential oils, which are made of natural ingredients and provide some type of aromatherapy.

As the pussy is a woman's most sensitive spot, make sure to use massage oil that won't cause any irritation down there. With that being said, I'd opt to use a lubricant instead, especially when you move to massaging the vagina. We use coconut oil to massage out bodies and when it comes to massaging her pussy I like to use ID Glide. My wife loves the feeling of this lubricant and believe me we have used many of them. It is so important that you find something that she likes and not something that you like. This lubricant is so soft and silky on her vagina.

Basically, you can choose among the following:

- Water-based lubricant

- Silicone-based lubricant

- Oil-based lubricant

- Natural lubricant

-

The water-based lubricant is usually the safest for the skin. Yet, it also dries up much quicker than others. Therefore, you would have to reapply it more often, which is quite a hassle.

Silicone-based lubes last much longer than water-based, so you can use them if you have them. ID Glide also makes a silicone-based lubricant.

Personally, I'd opt for the oil-based lubricant as it's very long-lasting. Also, it's the perfect time to use it! It's quite a picky type of lube.

Like it's REALLY good. But usually, you can't use it when wearing a condom or on some types of sex toys as it might rip the condom or ruin the toy so be careful if you planning to use a dildo during your massage.

So, it's usually left unused.

Now, you can make use of them for the massage as you'll only be using your hands.

Chapter 4

Starting The Erotic Massage Session

As we said mindfulness is key in giving a good massage. To start, you should have an intentional session with your lover for connecting.

Here's how:

Sit across from each other. You can do it cross-legged on the floor or by sitting on a chair facing each other.

Look directly at each other's eyes and hold some eye contact for at least 60 seconds.

Then synchronize your breaths slowly and deeply while maintaining eye contact.

Ask her if she has anything to say.

Show some gratitude to each other. After you are better connected lay her down and.

Warm Her Up With A Whole-Body Massage

A truly relaxing and effective pussy massage starts with a regular full-body massage. That means you don't lay her down and dive straight to the pussy from the get-go.

Warming up is always essential to ease the body into the massage.

You DON'T have to know everything or act like you know everything about giving a massage. I mean you are not a professional, unless you are. Since you're not a professional masseuse *(at least, you, the reader, are reading this guide now),* and that's totally okay.

You should go for showing her your love and the energy you have for her but putting it into your fingertips and hands and letting those travel into her body that way. Your body will naturally know what to do.

If you're an overachiever and perfectionist like me, you can check out some books or videos on to learn some basics of body massages.

Starting The Massage

Have your wife lie in a prone position or face down.

Begin to massage her back, neck, arms, thighs, calves, and feet in slow and long strokes.

Do this for at least about 10 to 15 minutes.

This is also a good point to start the communication. Ask if the pressure you are applying is okay, if she has any requests, and if it feels good or not.

Massaging Her Breasts

The breasts of a lady no matter what size they are may be a woman's most amazing erogenous zone on her body. Plus, they have muscles and nodes all around the area that could feel really relaxing for her when stimulated right. For some ladies like my wife, it gives her great pleasure AND sends her into a deep state of relaxation.

I like to at times position her hands above her head for easy access.

Then I cup the base of her breasts and rub it in a circular motion along the upper edges. I like to stop right below her armpits.

Then place your hands on her breastbone and work from the center of her chest to the sides of her body.

It's best to do one breast at a time to fully stimulate it.

Just slowly stroke along the breast tissue and knead through the knots you'll feel all across it. Doing so will promote blood flow and circulation in the breast.

When you see that her nipples are visually erect, you can also start stimulating them if you want to.

Lightly trace her areola, which is the pigmented darker area that surrounds the nipples with soft, feather-like touches.

When you move to finally touch her nipples, gently pinch from the root of the nipple. You can then switch from light pinching to hard squeezes.

I like to roll her nipples between my thumb and index finger. Another amazing move is to trace the figure out around her nipples.

Moving On To Massaging Her Thighs

This step often transitions from the regular full-body massage to the full-on pussy massage.

Start by doing long strokes from her inner thigh up to her vulva. This move often relaxes her pelvis for most ladies.

You should knead along the creases on her hips where you'll feel some knots. You can also knead these with the pad of your thumb by making small circles.

Ask her if she has any requests or if she wants you to get back and focus again on any other body parts. Then, if she wants you to proceed, you can move on to massaging her prize, the vulva.

How To Starting The Vulva Massage

Start by standing between her legs and placing both hands on her thighs. I like to pause at this time and take a moment to appreciate her genitals. Often, I will

26

bend over and smell them to take in the sweet aroma of her aroused honey pot. For I love the smell of my wife's pussy

You should also verbally express your adoration for its beauty. All women have a different looking pussy and all of them have their own beauty about it. Often times emotions and sensations can arise during the session. I like to place a flat palm on two parts. One is over the vulva area. And the other hand is over her heart. Stay in this post for at least 60 seconds before you move on to another technique.

Use this move to time and to synchronize your breaths.

Breathing is very important in a pussy massage. You and your girl should both breathe deeply, gathering air deep from your belly and then slowly letting it all out.

Get back to this pose any time she needs to take a break from the erotic action.

This should also be the ending pose as the session ends. Another reason to have this pose is to connect you and your lover's energies physically. The contact with her heart and vagina creates a bridge for your energies to travel from the heart and genitals.

It also aids in making your woman feel comforted and nurtured, which is really, really important. Making her feel safe, vulnerable, and revered at the same time is one of the key goals for an effective pussy massage.

Actually, Massaging Her Pussy

Now, you're finally ready to move on to the full-on pussy massage! There actually is no definite timeline on how long it should take. But if you want to have an estimate, you can do it for more or less 30 minutes.

Just Go Slow

Always remember to go slow for each technique, move, and step. There's no rush for a pussy massage.

In most of our sexual acts, we usually go fast to make our partners climax. Friction is what makes someone cum and so speed produces orgasms. But in a pussy massage, orgasm isn't the end goal as it's more for a healing touch. Still, she could orgasm from slow stimulations, which will sometimes feel more profound and intense to her.

So, what's the ideal pace? Twice slower than what you're thinking.

Be Attentive To How She Responds

In the next chapter, we'll give you the actual techniques for massaging her pussy. But there's no specific order or right or wrong way to go about it. Thus, you should be perceptive to her vocal and visual cues.

Things like her breathing could go fast or hitch if she's aroused. She might also show you some subtle body movements that will indicate if she's enjoying it or not enjoying a specific sensation.

Of course, you don't have to just keep on observing and guessing. As we've mentioned, the importance of communication should be established early on

Chapter 5

Great Pussy Massage Techniques

Palming A Pussy

You must avoid any type of direct stimulation of her clitorus at this time. Especially during this move. Instead, the primary purpose of this amazing technique is to simply warm up her vagina and get her insides to lubricate it.

You should position yourself in between her legs or at her side.

If you're positioned at her side:

Place the base of your palm at the bottom of the region of her vulva. And draw your palm up to her belly, letting your fingers trail along slowly behind it. It's also good to have your other hand follow the motions and trace the same path in one big continuous movement.

Alternate the strokes with one hand right after the other. It is quite amazing for her when you do this and never actually give her pussy lag time.

If you're positioned in between her legs:

Begin with your palm at the base of her vulva. And then draw your palm up from the vagina to her belly, but let your fingers lead the way this time.

Keep doing these strokes in an overlapping and alternating motion with your hands.

Cupping Her Vulva

This move is meant for grounding and easing her into the actual pussy massage. With an outstretched hand, just cup your hand over her whole vulva. Place your other hand on top of your outstretched hand. And gently press your hand into her vulva. Slowly, make a circling motion with your hand in a clockwise motion. You can also switch it up and go in a counterclockwise direction. Do this step for around 30 to 60 seconds. Then switch directions and do it for the same amount of time.

Light Stroking

Soft stroking for mindfulness using the least dominant finger—that is the ring finger. Simply stroke the soft inside groove of her outer labia with the pad of your ring finger. You can do this on one side at a time while allotting 30 to 60 seconds per side.

Then, just switch.

Light Pinching

This is a very good technique to stretch the skin that is around the vulva.

Do this by splaying your thumbs and fingers wide on opposite sides of the clitoral mound. Then gather the flesh by lightly squeezing the skin together. As you tug it lightly, make a rocking motion from side to side. This amazing motion is similar to pinching the skin but with less strength and a wider finger placement.

Pulling On The Lips

For this move use your thumbs and forefingers to "clip" the inner labia, that is the inner vaginal lips that look like petals jutting out in her vaginal opening. Please do this gently sir. You can lightly tug the inner labia to stretch it softly. Pull it from one side for around 5 seconds, then switch to the other side.

Release her lips and then repeat it all over again.

Direct Perineum Play

The perineum is that amazing spot of skin between the opening of her vagina and her anus. This spot has A LOT of nerve endings and holds a large amount of tension for most women. Stimulating this can be also arousing and pleasurable for your lady. Push the pad of your thumb into her perineum. Do this move in an acupressure style. Then alternate the pressure.

Using Deep Pressure

This is a healing technique that allows you to apply some deep pressure throughout her genitals while doing the move. This move is meant to be done slowly, giving your woman the feeling of focusing on her genitals, and it should be relaxing and arousing.

Use just the pad of both thumbs to trace lines starting from the area near her perineum, up and surrounding the vulva, and then up to the outer labia.

Massage a curved line up that goes past the clitoris. Then finish along the area that reaches her pubic hair. Do some tracing motions on both sides for several minutes.

Clit Caressing

This technique is amazing for most women. It is best to use it right before you go into penetration. Take careful note, that a pussy massage doesn't need to have type of penetration to be effective. Suppose she's not up for penetration, no problem. But it can be quite arousing for her anyway, so what if your partner might want some penetration—like finger-to-her pussy and or a cock to her pussy. You can quickly oblige her.

Another good move is using just your ring finger, lightly caress either side of the clitoris for a few minutes. Continue stroking up on top of the clit. You can stroke up and down it or in small circles around it.

Vary the pressure, strength, and speed you use as well. As you're stroking her clit, just place your other ring finger right at the vaginal opening.

You shouldn't put it inside yet Instead just set it right at the vaginal opening so she can FEEL it is there without putting it in. The suspense is a killer.

If It's Time, Go Ahead And Add Penetration

Again, as I have already said, this is a really OPTIONAL step. The first important thing before going to this step is to have her consent. So, please discuss beforehand what kind of a pussy massage you're going for. Going from the clit caressing technique, you can slowly insert just one finger into her pussy, preferably the ring finger. You may also use your middle finger as softly as you can.

You just don't want to go in *too* deep—yet. So, go ahead and stop at your first knuckle. And make sure you do it SLOWLY.

Then, make little circles gently around the vaginal opening. You can just focus on this for about 30 to 60 seconds. While doing this, you may also want to stimulate her clit.

Massage The G-Spot.

Now some women like their G-spot to be stimulated; and others don't. But most of the time, they do. As the massage progresses it can be very arousing for her, and your lover might want you to go all the way. That means she may want to squirt or ejaculate. Otherwise, it might make her feel unsatisfied as her vagina isn't really stimulated.

Leaving her feeling frustrated from a pussy massage session is the exact opposite of what you want to accomplish here.

So, again, it should be HER choice. Ask her and listen to each other well.

In case you don't know the G-spot is a spongy nub that is located in the upper vaginal wall in the front. It's not too deep—only around 1 to 3 inches inside. Please remember that it's different from woman to woman. So, using your finger is sufficient enough.

How To Correctly Stimulate Her G-Spot

Just curl your finger slightly into like the C-shape. Keep your finger's pose loose and light. Then slowly do a come-hither motion with your finger, applying a dragging sensation on the G-spot.

Another variation is to put some pressure on the G-spot by pressing the G-spot for 10 to 20 seconds. Then release and then repeat it again. Do these strokes for several minutes. You may ask her if she wants you to raise the intensity by increasing the speed or pressure you are using on her G-spot. With these techniques, your lady could experience wave after wave of intense orgasms with all the different combination of stimulations you are using. Her climax could feel very sexual or a more gentle and nurturing massage sensation that feels pleasurable from deep inside her being.

Bring A Sex Toy Into The Session

Adding a sex toy like a vibrator can provide much more stimulation than your fingers can ever do on their own. The ones with low intensity are perfect for teasing. And a toy you can put on your finger is a great way to give her vibrations and stimulation from the ribbed textures.

Be Open For Requests

This is the next step after:

If she doesn't want penetration, or if she said yes to penetration.

Before ending the pussy massage session, ask her if she has any requests.

For example, she might want you to repeat some pussy massage techniques that you have already done. Sometimes, she might ask you to use your tongue to massage her instead of your fingers. Oh yes, I love to eat my wife's pussy. And she might even request for you to fuck her hard. Again, there should be no pressure for her to want it. But if she does, then it's a very welcome bonus, isn't it?

As you're doing the discussion with her, don't stop massaging her pussy. Continue massaging her pussy slowly and gently.

Always End Each Session With Some Tender Loving Care

Ending the pussy massage heavily lies in her decision. The erotic session could end by you making love to her. Or it could end with some cuddling and talking about the whole experience. Either way, it's up to what she's in for.

This is why it's an unconditional act, after all it's a session that is just for her wants and her needs.

When you end the session, place both palms back on her vulva and heart and pause for a moment.

The last step is to always sit back to talk and share your intimacy of the experience and what you learned from it.

As with giving a tantric massage, you can cement the sensual bonding experience by conversing about your deep realizations and unearthing emotions you felt during the session. If it's the first time for you and your lover to do a pussy massage, skip any type of sex and penetration.

This makes the practice even more effective because you and your lady can feel more grounded and realize that not all intimate sex acts should always lead to sexual escalation. Doing any stimulation or contact with her genitals that ends with sex could feel like you're going the habitual route.

Skipping it for at least for the first session gives a rarity to the experience.

Your lady will also feel like she's treasured, especially as the entire session is really ONLY for her.

A pussy massage may sound like a lot of work. But trust me it's really worth it because it encompasses sexual experience in the physical realm. You can also connect emotionally and sensually, which is really rare and valuable these days in our natural lives.

A sexy massage carries a whole load of other benefits. And that's why tantric practices are always worth exploring.

Just Give Her Some Aftercare

Once you're finally done, follow her lead. She might want to fuck. She might want to grab you, and push you down on the bed, and tell you it's your turn. Or she might just want to cuddle.

I've heard of women feeling emotional after a pussy massage, so be ready for that, too. If she feels weird or needs to cry or whatever, just hold her and be there for her. And show her how much you love her. Understand that it's probably a good thing - it means you have put her body through some really intense pleasure. Give her something special.

I know it's kind of funny to write a quick and sexy guide to something that it can easily last over an hour. But I really do want to spread the word about this great practice that most women will absolutely lover their husband to do for them. Pussy massages are a great way for couples to reconnect, to do something sexual even on those low libido days, or just for the sake of feeling good.

So, give her a special night. Tell her to lie down and relax, give yourself plenty of time to massage her right, and make her feel amazing.

Chapter 6

Adding Some Amazing Anal Massage Techniques

Unlike a pussy massage an Anal massage stimulates a woman both mentally and emotionally. For most ladies it's also a huge turn-on as anything to do with anal or ass play is seen as "taboo" or "forbidden." It can be fun to do in the bedroom. The role of taboo and forbidden acts in a woman's psyche is extremely underestimated, as women have a totally different attitude when come to sex than most men do.

And anal massage is one of the best ways to get a woman to explore her deep, hidden desires.

With all that being said anal massage can be a little tricky to get started. Although I must admit is one of the most erotic things a couple can do together is to massage each other's anus. After you learn how to do it, soon if will become something that you almost can't do without as it feels that good. If you are wondering where to start at giving your spouse an anal massage? The techniques below can be used by both men and women. As long as there are two willing participants, you can use the techniques for hours and hours of fun. Now let's get into how you should prepare for an anal massage properly, and then we'll move onto some naughty techniques!

Here's the techniques I use, and they work for me, so I'm sure they will work for you as well.

I like to start out my slowing by drawing big soft circles around the rim of my wife's butthole. This erotic practice alone actually builds up anticipation while setting some distance so that she doesn't feel too overwhelmed by an all-out assault on her butthole. After some time, you have to determine for yourself how long that is, then you can move into making a big circular motion around their anus with little loops drooping in between. It's such a subtle change of movement that it will probably add a tickling sensation to them and wake up the nerve endings that are located all around the anus.

You can also add a little variety if you like by stroking their anus gently using just one finger. Basically, you're lightly flicking your finger from their perineum (which is that patch of skin that is located at the base of a man's cock or between the vaginal opening and her anus) all across the anus. Now again make the same stroking motions, but this time add some more fingers. Keep it to around three fingers at the most, then stroke up to down to cover a larger area.

Another variation of this that you can use is simply rubbing the anus directly. Instead of stroking it in one single direction though, rub it up and down to heighten the sensations. If your lover enjoys it, you can cover a bigger zone using three fingers instead of just one. To amplify the sensation even more now start using both hands. Stroke down going in different directions using both hands, sort of like you're opening up the anus for further exploration. Still using both of your hands together split their buttocks and gently thumb and massage the area all around the anus with both thumbs, moving your way up. This move is sometimes called the Lumberjack move. This is more of a warm-up move, as you're not actually inserting any fingers into her yet. Once you've applied some lube to your hands and on her ass cheeks, simply put your hands together like you're praying and rub them in between her cheeks with a sawing motion.

Be sure when you are starting out to go slowly and softly, and then later on as she's more comfortable you can start increasing the speed and pressure that you apply. You can also vary the speed to tease her a little as well. This move will get her good and used to the sensation around that area and get her nicely warmed up for the more hardcore techniques later on like Thumb Twiddling. I know this all is strange sounding, but it is actually quite simple.

You want to place both hands like a fist between her ass cheeks and spread them apart with your knuckles. At this point, your thumbs should be right above her anus. Slowly move them around in a circular motion, being sure to smoothly rub the outside of her anus. Much like you did at first when you were rubbing her with three fingers.

Again, be sure to use plenty of lube. You can of course increase the speed and intensity as you go on and she's more comfortable.

Now you can at this time extend to other erogenous zones as well. For example, the groin area that is located behind her thighs. If it feels ticklish and sensitive, reaching these areas will have a much bigger effect on them. Please don't ignore what's right in front of you. While your hands are doing the massage, you can also multitask and even include your mouth and tongue in on the erotic action if you are feeling a little kinky. You can even suck his penis or lick her vagina while massaging their anus. I absolutely love it when my wife multitasks on my special parts. I believe that your lover will feel like it's the best day of their lives.

Okay it's finally time to talk about graduating from anal massage to anal fingering.

If the goal of your anal massage is to get your partner ready for some amazing anal fingering, then do the techniques we have already mentioned beforehand and move on to these erotic moments with your hands. Massaging their anus area gently like the above steps can help relax them while turning them on as well. The more aroused and relaxed they are, the easier it will be for your finger to actually penetrate them without any pain at all. The first time I thumbed my wife's ass I was fucking her in doggie, and she went crazy bucking me like a bronco and I knew I had found something that she absolutely loved. So, I began sticking a lubed finger in her anus when I was finger fucking her as well and she came so hard she filled my hand up with a puddle of cum. Now she begs me to fuck her ass with a finger or two while we are playing with each other.

I guess what I am trying to say is that there is no necessary switch you have to flip to go from the massage to the fingering. Just listen to your lover's reactions and assess if they're ready and even wanting it. But please do it gently, and of course with well lubricated fingers. Don't just poke your finger into their ass out of nowhere. You may also ask them or even inform them that you are ready to start fingering their ass and are they ready.

Anyway, you're not going to put your finger in that tight hole immediately. First, you will have to put more pressure on the anus and massage it until you can slowly get your finger into the anus up to the first knuckle.

The more anal lube you use, the better. Reapply it often and be as liberal as you can. More lubrication back there definitely feels infinitely better.

For most ladies did you know that "Two Holes Are Better Than One." Now it's time to double penetrate your lover! What we're talking about is fingering both her pussy and ass at the same time. As this can be quite overwhelming for her to say the least. I recommend doing this after she's used to the anal fingering from the previous techniques we mentioned. Then while you're still fingering her ass, take your other hand and insert a finger or two into her vagina. By this point, there's no need to be so gentle on her pussy if she's like my wife, she's probably drenching wet from all the previous techniques earlier. We call this "two in the pink and one in the stink."

You can probably even start off with two fingers. So, by now you've got two fingers in her pussy and one in her ass fingering her at a moderate pace. While you're doing this your woman is probably moaning like crazy, experiencing new heights of pleasure she's never felt before. At this point sometimes I like to switch it up. I do everything I can to keep our love life from becoming routine. I'll either add my tongue to the mix which is called "rimming" and eat her ass out completely or I'll double up. That's amazing at times if we are planning on having anal sex later. No, we're not done yet – there's yet another level to anal massage or fingering, whatever you want to call it. This one might be a bit challenging due to physical limitations and probably is not for everyone.

Bluntly speaking, we're going to attempt to insert two fingers up the ass. It's going to take a lot of patience, and lube. A LOT of lube.

Similar when you were first trying to insert your first finger up there, it's going to feel tight going really slow allowing her time to adjust because it is tight and uncomfortable for most ladies at first. So please be patient and don't be discouraged if it takes a long time or if it comes to the point where she's too uncomfortable to continue. You can always try next time. It took us several tries over a period of weeks, because my fingers are quite thick. Size 16 ring finger. Anyways, when you've finally managed to get two fingers in that tight hole, be really careful. Slowly move them in and out and pay attention to her reaction. You can then try bending your finger to stimulate the walls of the rectum and vaginal membrane. It can be just too painful for some ladies, and in that case, one finger is likely adequate. It's all about her pleasure and not your accomplishments, never forget that.

In case your wife really enjoys it, you can really explore with this and even try to insert even more fingers. However, if she is a non-professional at anal sex, it's highly unlikely she can handle more than one or two fingers up her ass. Nonetheless, one or two fingers is all it takes to feel really good for most ladies. Probably the best lube for anal play is silicone-based lubricants because they tend to be slippery and wetter feeling. Of course, water-based lubes also work fine.

But silicone lubes are thicker, last longer, and glide more easily. These are features you'd want when you are having erotic butt play. We like to use a cherry-flavored type of anal lube if we are going to do analingus on one another during our anal play session.

Almost 100 % of the time we use an anal douche beforehand, so we aren't worried about any poop making a cameo appearance in our anal playground.

We have also found when we are using a water-based lube, we also use a latex glove or finger cot to make our cleanup much easier. Please don't be afraid of funky smells on your hand or finger afterwards. Each body has its own essence of smells, regardless of how clean or fresh the anus is. So, it's totally natural to have a few little brown streaks and smells. As far as taste goes a clean anus tastes a little metallic and that's about it, really not too bad.

Another thing to never forget is to never, ever double dip. That is when you touch the anus with a finger, we should never move to touch the vagina with that same finger. I may be okay to do in porno movies but not so wise in real life. At least wash your hands first, Switching lanes will introduce fecal bacteria to the vagina, leading to possible urinary tract infection, or even a UTI, for some women. Also, as I said you don't have to worry much about poop. The poop is high up in her bowels, and not really in the rectum until moments before it is ready to be expelled from the body. That is unless you have really long fingers, you're not likely to reach that far up inside her. It's quite normal to feel like you're pooping when your anus is being filled up and stimulated with something. But you're not actually pooping, I promise.

Also, for some people your butt muscles and anus can feel a little sore after some intense anal play. Just go get a warm bath with some Epsom salts, that will definitely help.

If you really want to do this as a married couple and you are having problems with insertion at first just, try and try again. You can't go from zero to three fingers in one session with patience, believe it or not. It's all about relaxation on the receiver's part. So, it's essential to go gradually and slowly. Along the way, you can also apply everything you've learned from past sessions to make the whole erotic experience feel more pleasurable for both parties. Don't you think it's time to start exploring the backdoor with a great anal massage. It's a great addition to a pussy massage.

If it's your first step to dip your toes into anal play—great for assessing if it feels good to you without worrying about any penetration yet.

This is really one of those things that you have to try for yourself before deciding if it's for you or not. You might think it's a bit too freaky and out there for you to try, but once trying you will actually get addicted! So, don't be afraid to try. Most Woman have some kind of secret taboo to various kinks and fetishes you would've never imagined and are more open-minded than you thought.

Bringing up anal massage and fingering and similar things to your wife, and then of course trying it can be a great way to improve your relationship. The taboo and forbidden aspect of anal play, along with just how good it actually feels, is a great thing to add to your bedroom repertoire.

I warn you though once you start incorporating anal fingering and other types of anal play into your sex life, there's no turning back.

What My Wife Says About A Pussy Massage

I once got the incredible experience of a pussy-massage each night for a whole week. As a woman, if you have never had one, I highly recommend it sister! During that week I discovered places in myself that I didn't know existed. I got a deepening in my connection with my husband and learned how to be the receiver of pleasure for the moment. It is an amazing process, and I hope that I can try to convey to you the profound power of this sacred sexual practice so that you too can learn how to have this kind of experience.

The ancients call it a "Yoni" (pronounced yo-knee) massage which is nothing more than another word for vagina. But its true meaning goes far beyond the physical realm. The word was actually first mentioned in the "Kama Sutra", and its meaning is loosely translated as "sacred altar" or "sacred space." When it is spoken of in tantric terms, the "Yoni" becomes the sacred doorway to the Goddess, as an aspect of the divine. This was a place to worship, and the goal of the Yoni massage it just that, the man is to worship the sacred temple that is known as the "Yoni."

The feminine is all about pleasure, and this massage helps a woman tap into and understand her deep connection to her bodily pleasure. This massage isn't so much sexual as it is sensual, it is designed to promote relaxation and openness in a woman.

Orgasm isn't the goal, although orgasm may definitely and probably will occur during a pussy massage, and it may be more intense and expansive and more deeply satisfying than all other orgasms. The person giving a pussy massage is a witness to the beauty of all that is feminine. You, sir as the massager, are worshiping at her sacred temple known as her "Yoni." Remembering this and connecting to the "Great Feminine" through your lover throughout the massage will make it a way more powerful experience for both of you. Touch her as you would touch a goddess—that is with reverence, awe, respect, and great love.

One nice thing to do is take a bath together beforehand it is a beautiful ritual to partake in before a pussy massage. We did every night in preparation. You can start your process of worshipping her long before you touch her pussy. Use essential oils in the bath water such as lavender. It is known as a wonder relaxer. Wash her hair for her. Dry her body off with a warmed towel after the bath and moisturize her skin. Make sure you both go to the bathroom before starting, as you won't want to have to interrupt the flow if one of you has to use the bathroom.

We set up a massage room to do the massages in with a heated massage table. You need a quiet, preferably dim space, with a bed, or a futon mattress on the floor, or even pillows, or a massage table. We lit scented candles. You can drape a sheet over them, in case you spill any oil. The temperature in the room should be a little warmer than normal because you are both going to be nude during the whole massage, so you may want to turn up the heat a little. Lighting many candles in the room also helps generate heat, as well as giving the room a soft glow, especially if you use coconut oil on her skin. You will want to make sure that you have an open time frame where you won't be disturbed, preferably a few hours. Our kids we moved out. Remember to turn off all of your phones, and if you live with others, you can even put a "Do Not Disturb" sign on the door.

Music is really good to set the mood but be sure it's something where all of the tracks are appropriate. There's nothing so jarring as a radical piece of music suddenly playing when you're trying to relax. Make sure your CD player has a "repeat" function, so you don't have to stop to push "play" again and again. We actually use massage CD's made for giving massages.

These are sensual delights and will help soften a woman into her feminine nature. Have soft, cut up juicy fruits around, especially exotic ones like mangoes and papaya, but even peaches and pears and banana's work in a pinch. Feed her with your fingers, let the juices run down her chin. This flow will encourage her to flow you know where.

Your lubricants and oils should be somewhere within easy reach. Try to get spill proof bottles and use plastic rather than glass. Knocking over a bottle of massage oil and breaking it as it makes a huge mess goes a long way toward ruining the sensual mood! Now I'll let my husband take it from here.

When you are giving this massage, you should remind your lover that their communication with you is key. Make sure that they feel comfortable making some requests and comments. She should know that this is about her comfort and pleasure. This alone can be a difficult practice for some women, and you can often encourage her by asking "Is this too hard?" or "Is the temperature, okay?" just to get her into the swing of things.

The first thing you should do is breathe together. Breathing is the way we make love with our lover. Look into each other's eyes and breathe together, deep into your belly. You should be sitting face-to-face or even standing, if you prefer. You can hold hands, or hold onto each other, whatever you want and feels good to you both.

The massage also begins with her lying on her back, usually with something under her hips to lift her up a little. Maybe a pillow, just cover it with a towel. She can place a pillow under her head if she wants to, or not, whichever is more comfortable for her. Make sure she is relaxed and truly comfortable before you begin, because she is going to be in this position for a long time.

If you are doing this on a bed you should sit between the woman's legs, cross-legged. Tell her to bend her knees slightly and then let them fall open for you. You can also position her legs for her if you like. You should continue looking into her eyes and breathing with her. Remind her, often, of her breathing. If you find she is holding her breath, you can place your hand on her lower belly and remind her to breathe from that space, and to "fill her belly" with her breath. Practice this a few times before you actually begin.

Pussy massage begins with a slow, sensual massage of the other parts of her body. Massage her feet, legs, belly, breasts, and her arms. This a long, slow process my friend. Look at the feminine form that is laying in front of you, as you breathe her in—think about her as your goddess. Worship her femininity with your hands, and your eyes as you breathe the aroma of her femininity. I don't know about you, but I love the smell of my wife's essence. Advance the massage slowly toward her inner thighs and pelvis, until she is breathing deeply from her belly, and her body has no more tension and is fully relaxed.

Then, and only then, should you approach her pussy. This is a sacred act, and a powerful one. You should ask her permission to enter her temple. You can simply say the words, "May I touch your pussy baby?" or you can more formally ask, "May I touch your sacred spot?" She may giggle, or smile at you. Some women may actually get tears in her eyes. Most women have never had their bodies held in such regard and worshipped in such a way, and any reaction is normal. Just take it in stride, whatever it is.

If she gives you her permission to touch her, and she will, simply pour a small quantity of very good quality massage oil or water-based lubricant on the mound of her pussy, just so that it drips down over the vulva or the outer lips. The quality of the oil is so very important. This area of the body is very sensitive, and the skin can get raw quickly if the oil isn't high quality. You should plan to spend a great deal of time here, just rubbing the oil into the vulva. Use slow, steady motions. You can cup her entire pussy with your hand and massage it that way as well. Then focus on the outer lips: squeeze each lip between your thumb and forefinger, stroking up and down the entire length.

Remember, too, to ask her what she is feeling—is it too hard, too soft? Too fast, too slow? Let her pleasure be your guide. You don't need to have a conversation and probably shouldn't. But definitely keep communicating during the massage. Look into her eyes and keep breathing with her.

Next, do the same motion over her inner lips, squeezing each one between your thumb and forefinger, stroking up and down the length. Spend as much time as you need here—this isn't about rushing through it. Her vagina is a sacred space, and you are making your way through it, tenderly exploring it completely. Worship every soft, delicate fold of her pussy as you massage her.

When you do this her clitoris should be stroked gently, first with clockwise pattern, then counterclockwise circles. You should then squeeze it between thumb and index finger, and gently pull on it. You should continue to stimulate her clitoris in these slow, easy circles. She will probably become very aroused during this process but continue to encourage her to relax and breathe.

When you have spent your time here, you should move on to the entrance of her temple—it is time to enter her pussy. Again, you should ask her for permission, in whatever way feels most comfortable for you to say. "May I enter your pussy sweetheart?" is fine, as well as "May I enter your sacred space?" Gently insert one finger some women like my wife prefer two, you can ask which she likes slowly into her cunt. If she prefers one, use the middle finger of your right hand. If she prefers two, use your middle and index fingers.

Gently explore and massage the inside of your wife's pussy with your finger(s). This is a massage, remember that, and while you *are* penetrating her, this isn't about simulating her to climax. This is about truly discovering what she feels like inside her sweetness, reveling in every glorious inch of her flesh, and allowing her to feel your worship of her while she experiences the pleasurable sensations of her own body.

Explore all the textures of her vagina, the smoothness, the softness, the bumps, with your finger(s). Take it a fraction of an inch at a time. If you come up against spots that are painful and too tight, stop moving, but continue to press your fingers there. Women often carry years of pain, frustration, and trauma locked up tight inside their pussy and this massage can help release those if you are patient and gentle with her. You may be surprised if she starts to cry—whatever her reaction is, it's okay. This is about her releasing, and letting things flow. Even her strong emotions—like fear, anxiety, or even joy—could come up. Encourage her to let them flow freely through her as you keep massaging the inner walls of her temple. She may also experience some tingling or heat in those places where there once was tension. This is normal as well. Keep breathing together.

If you have been using just your middle finger, simply insert the finger between the pinky and the middle finger and, with your palm facing up, put them as far as they will go inside of her pussy. Now, curl your fingers in a "come here" type of gesture—crooking them back towards the palm. This is the area known as the G-spot (which is "sacred spot" in Tantra practices). It can be very sensitive, and it feels different from the vaginal walls. It's really soft and spongy to the touch. It's about the size of a postage stamp for most ladies. You will know you have found it because most women suddenly feel an urge to urinate when it is first stimulated. Or some may experience a kind of burning sensation. And again, some woman find it immediately very pleasurable. Continue focusing here on this spot, varying the speed and pressure to her liking. Remember to keep asking her for feedback about how you are doing and what she is feeling.

You can use your other hand, or the thumb of your right hand, to begin to stimulate her clitoris. You want to begin to awaken her to an even higher state of arousal. You can also, if she is willing, and a little kinky insert your pinky of your right hand into her anus. Please don't do this unless you already know she enjoys anal stimulation. During a pussy massage isn't the time to experiment with first time anal play! Experience the power of that moment together, breathe it into your bellies. You are worshipping the mystery she is, as woman of femininity.

Continue massaging her this way until she actually asks you to stop. For most woman like my wife during this action she may orgasm, either clitorally or vaginally, or some combination of them both. If she doesn't tell you to stop, then by all means don't. Many women can learn to have multiple orgasms using this technique. Keep reminding her to breathe from her belly and remember to breathe with her. You can use your other hand to press her womb, as a reminder. You can also use your other hand to massage her breasts, or her belly, or yes, her clitoris. You shouldn't, however, use your other hand for self-stimulation. You may have an erection—this is normal. Use that energy to focus on your woman in front of you, as you pour into her the passion and love and reverence you are feeling with your hands. It is a powerful gift you can give your wife.

You should only stop massaging when she tells you to stop. At that time, slowly and gently take your hands away. Thank her for the opportunity to worship her pussy, and then you can hold each other, kiss and cuddle if you like. If you are going to transition into some other form of sexual contact, Then I would recommend a break of some kind, Maybe go to the bathroom, or go to another room to continue. That is if you want to keep the pussy massage about worshipping her as a goddess, and don't want to diminish it in any way.

If you do pussy massages over a period of time, a woman can learn a new level of trust and intimacy and even a deeper connection to her body. Pussy massage can release layers of tension and allow a previously non-orgasmic woman to become orgasmic, or even to learn how to have multiple orgasms. Just remember, it is all about entering the temple of her divine femininity—so treat her with reverence, deep love, respect, and honor her for the great mystery that she is. If you do this correctly, you may find that the rewards are immeasurable.

Other Books By Thomas Kane

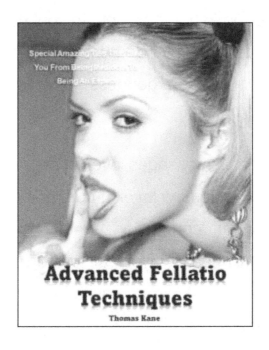

Advanced Fellatio Techniques

Some people wonder themselves, should I suck or not! That is the question? The truth is even though it's called a ******* there really is no blowing involved in it at all. And for the wife that really wants to please her husband there is no better thing then to pull off giving him a mind blowing *******. You know one that curls his toes and has him yelling your name as he's filling your mouth up with his love juice. I can safely say my husband is addicted to my mouth. Mainly because I know how to use my tongue, lips and throat just at the right time. That's what giving amazing ******** is all about timing. When you know how to do this or lick there or even went to swallow him down, you're on your way.

You bought this book probably because you already know how to give him ******** but you want to know how to do it better. Well sister, you bought the right book. These are some of the advanced techniques you will learn.

- some improved penis swallowing techniques

- how to really use that amazing tongue of yours

- how to really **** ****** a penis

- how to stop gagging all the time

- how to leave in breastless and begging for more

- the proper way to use your hands and so much more

Get a copy today and learn everything you need to know about pleasuring your man with your mouth some of the techniques go from mild to wild and I know he will be pleased when you use them on him. So tonight sit down on the couch take his shirt off, unzip his zipper and pull his boxers down and send him to orgasm heaven.

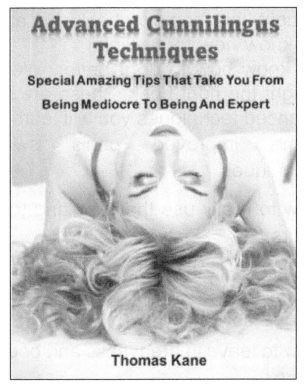

Advance Cunniligus Techniques

This is the true guidebook for giving your woman amazing oral sex.

Did you know that only 25% of all women achieve orgasms from sexual intercourse alone. Knowing this important fact makes this book a priceless resource for you. This is a step-by-step guide in how to give your woman the amazing oral pleasure she craves.

These advanced techniques you will learn will in fact give her stronger, and more intense orgasms.

This is next level stuff Sir. You see sex is a lot like a cake and all of the ingredients alone don't really taste that good. But when you mix them together right, they taste fantastic. And great cunnilingus it's just one of those ingredients.

In this book you will learn.
- How to give her multiple O's
- How to really give her a fantastic clitoral massage
- Advanced cunnilingus techniques that will make her scream
- How to really get yourself ready to eat her pussy
- And many more advanced techniques

So, do you want to leave her shaking in pleasure to the very core? Do you want to give her the most amazing pleasure she's ever had with just your mouth? If you use these techniques right, she will be screaming your name, squirting in your face and grabbing the back of your head as she squeezes her legs together in pleasure.

You will see her face get flush, with ecstasy all because of what you're doing with your mouth. So, if you want to give her mind-blowing orgasms with only your mouth and fingers and make her scream then get this book today! Beware, reading this book will teach you how to decode your wife's body!

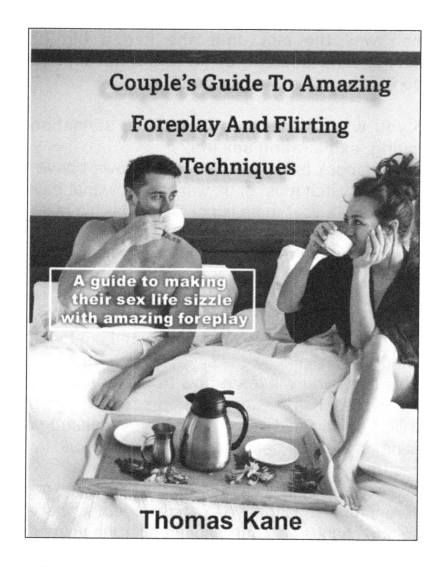

Couples guide to foreplay and flirting

DON'T JUST MAKE LOVE, BUT HAVE CRAZY, PASSATIONATE, TEAR EACH OTHER'S CLOTHES OFF SEX!!!!!!!

When was the last time she had a big hard sausage for breakfast, or he had a hot breakfast taco before getting out to bed?

Do you want to have an incredible, sensational, exciting, exhilarating sex life?
Then this book is for you! The great news I have for you today is that most of us want to know that having great sex with your mate is not an impossible feat.

But the truth is any couple can have a lot of fun in the bedroom that will most certainly lead to mind-blowing orgasms!

Most of us already have the basic ingredients to make it all happen. We just need to know how to use them correctly. Or should I say how to blend them together properly.

In this book you will learn how to make your willing partner who has a desire for more have greater passion as you add some skillful techniques to your routine that will definitely rock their world with pleasure.

Since every couple is unique, we have included many different fun things that you can do together to shake it up and change your marriage bed for the better.

That's why you bought this book right so you could make your marriage better. So, if your goal is to give your mate the best orgasm of their life you know one that shakes their body curls their toes and has them moaning your name like a howling dog then a little foreplay might be all you need. Get a copy today and find out how to make your marriage bed a better experience for the both of you. **Get A Copy Today!**

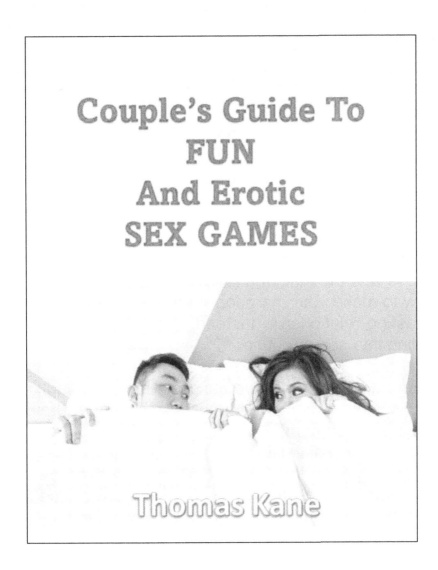

Couples Guide To Fun And Erotic Sex Games

DOES YOUR BEDROOM EXPERIENCE NEED A LITTLE SPICE?

If the answer to that question is yes, then adding some sex games may be the antidote to your boredom.

Don't let your marriage become boring and routine! Change things up and bring something new to the marriage bed. Author Thomas Kane has don't just that with some great ideas and plans.

I mean when was the last time you actually tried something new in the bedroom? Or are you just simply stuck in a missionary or doggie rut? Did you know that there are several studies out there that show that playing games with someone strengthens the relationship of the couple? It build togetherness and more intimate closeness.

That's why the main focus of this book is to teach you how to make your marriage burn brighter and make it a lasting relationship. Instead of just fizzling out and fading into some routine.

This book has dozens of ideas separated into eight different categories for you to use. There's enough fun in this book to keep any couple busy for months having fun in the bedroom.

Even if you're satisfied with your marriage and sex life today, I believe this book could make it even better. As you invite the love of your life to have a little fun and play together in bed.

Why not act like young people again and have fun in bed!!!!

When you both become more adventurous in your sex life it's very fun. Get a copy today!

Made in the USA
Las Vegas, NV
03 October 2024

96242485R10046